BYE BYE PACIFIER

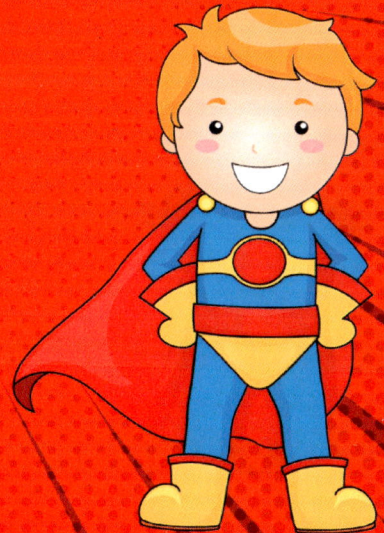

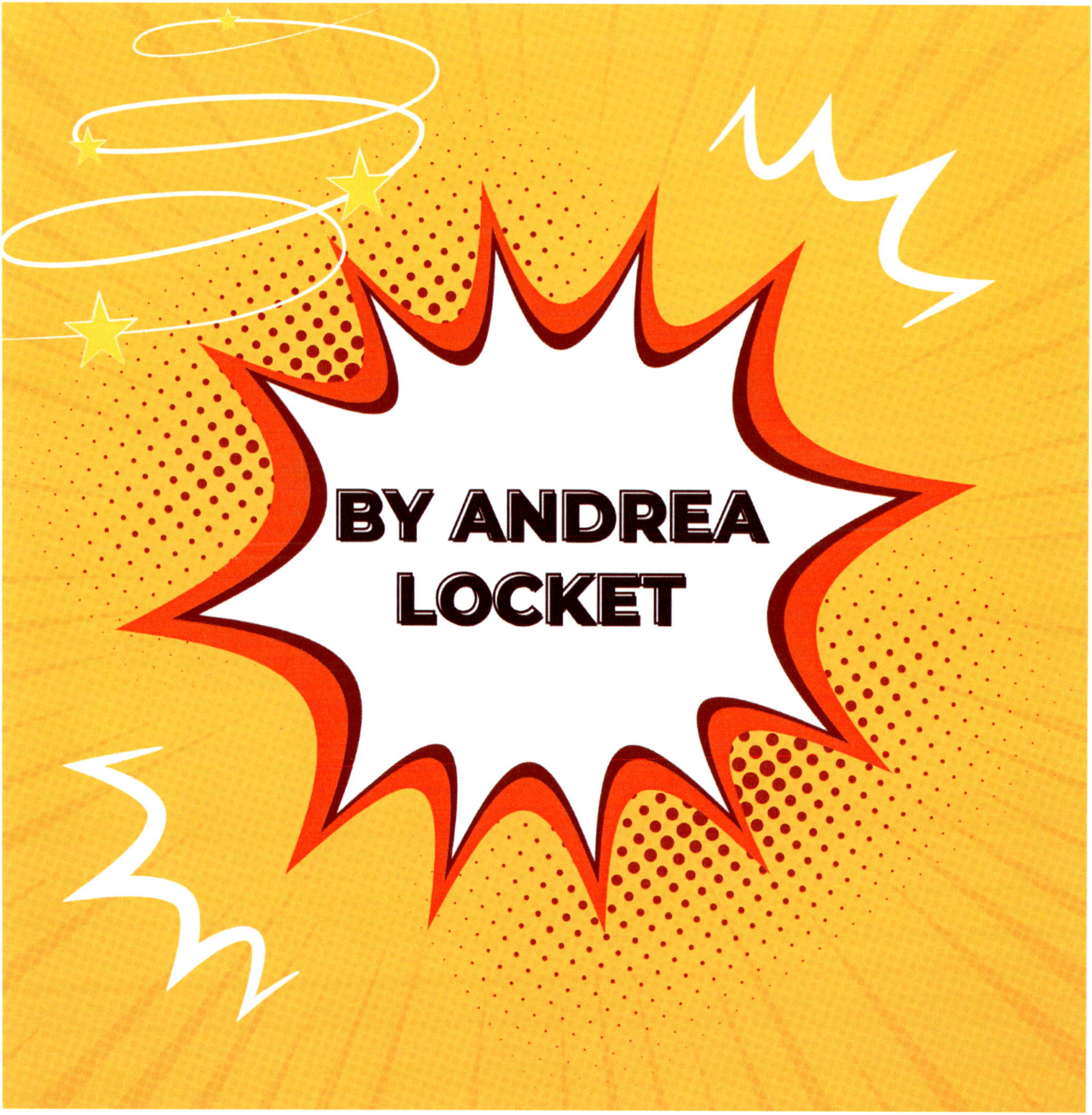
BY ANDREA
LOCKET

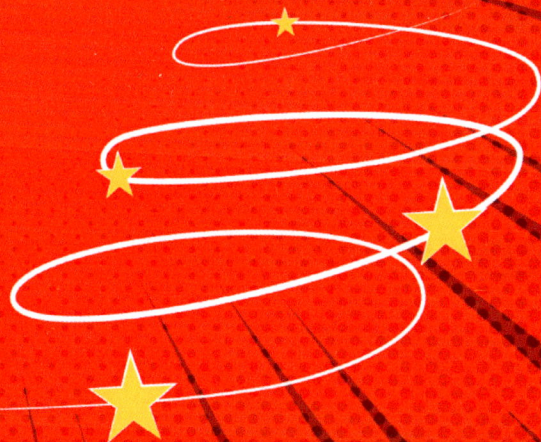

MEET JAMES - HE LOVES TO DRESS UP AS A SUPERHERO

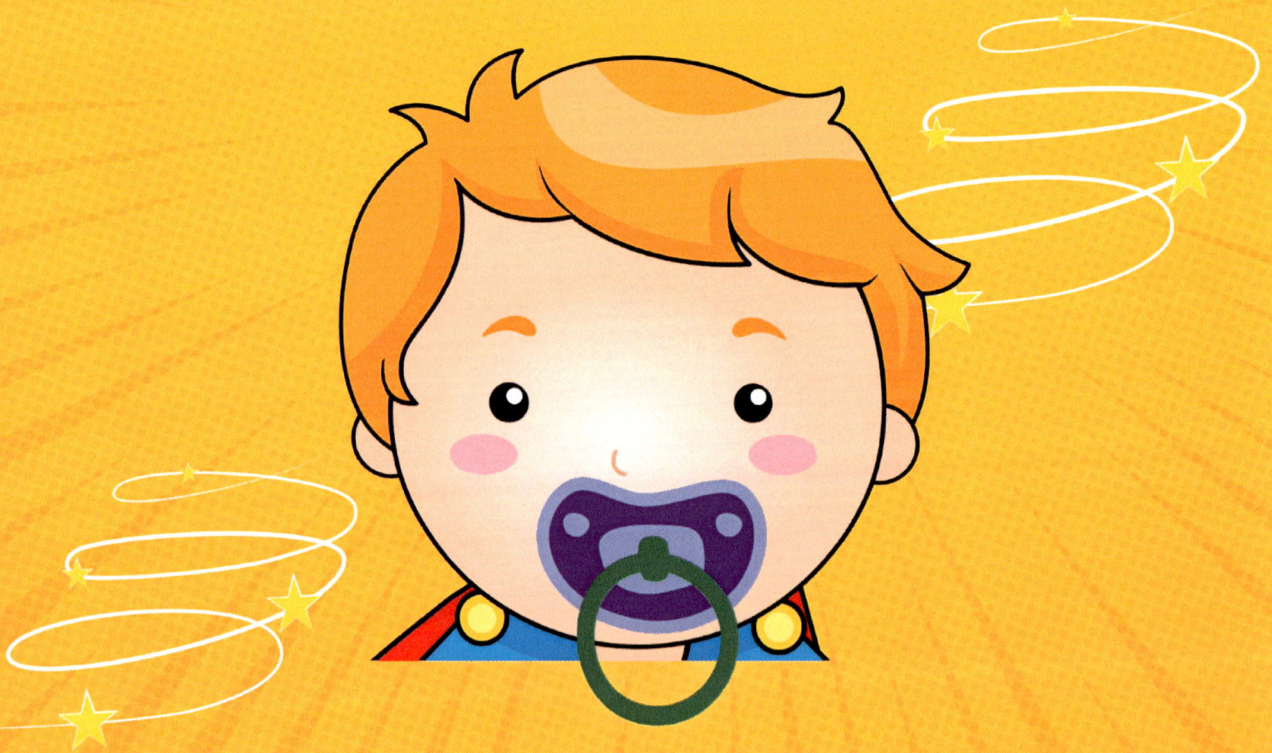

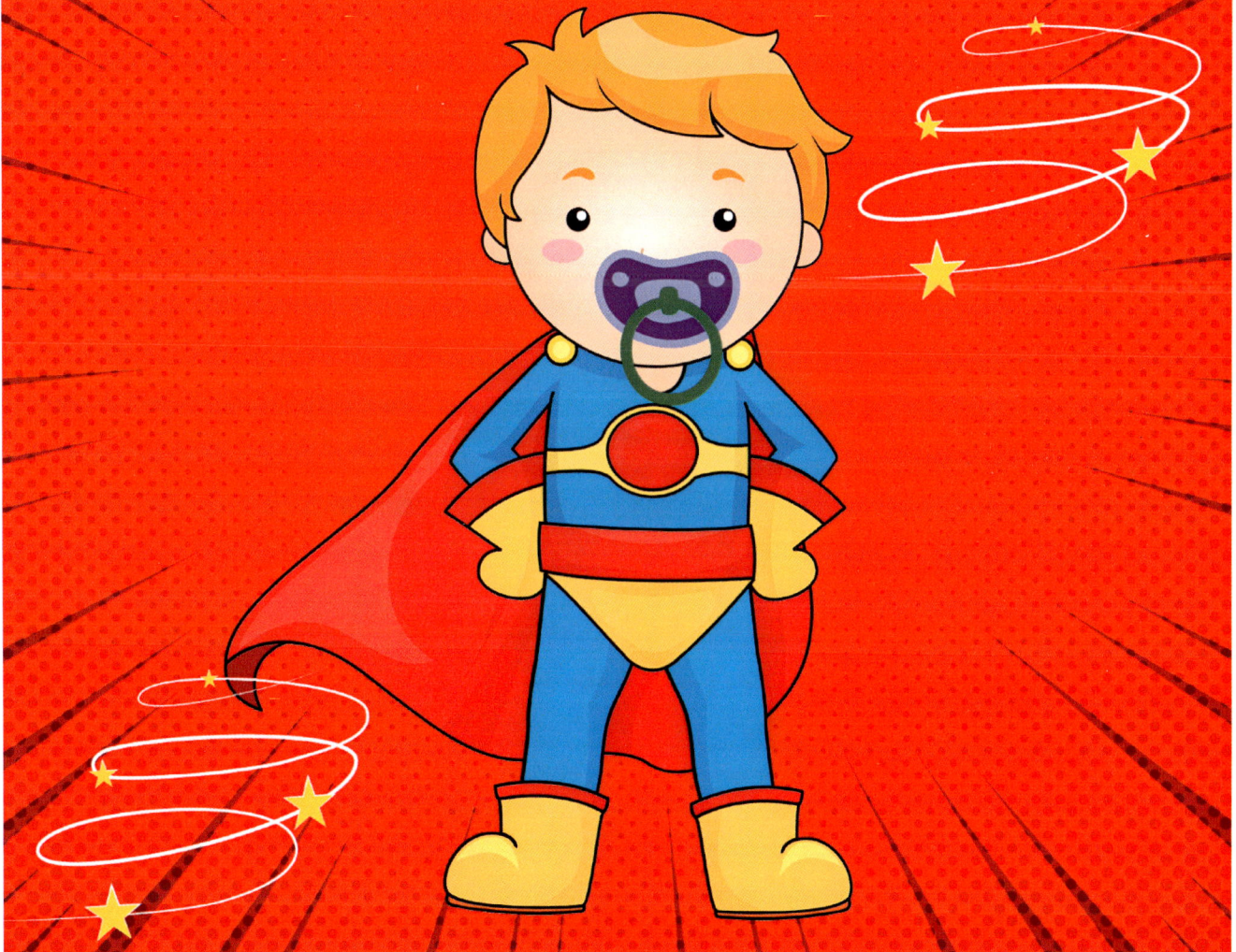

THIS IS HIS FAVORITE SUPERHERO COSTUME

BLUE SUIT

RED BELT

RED CLOAK

YELLOW BOOTS

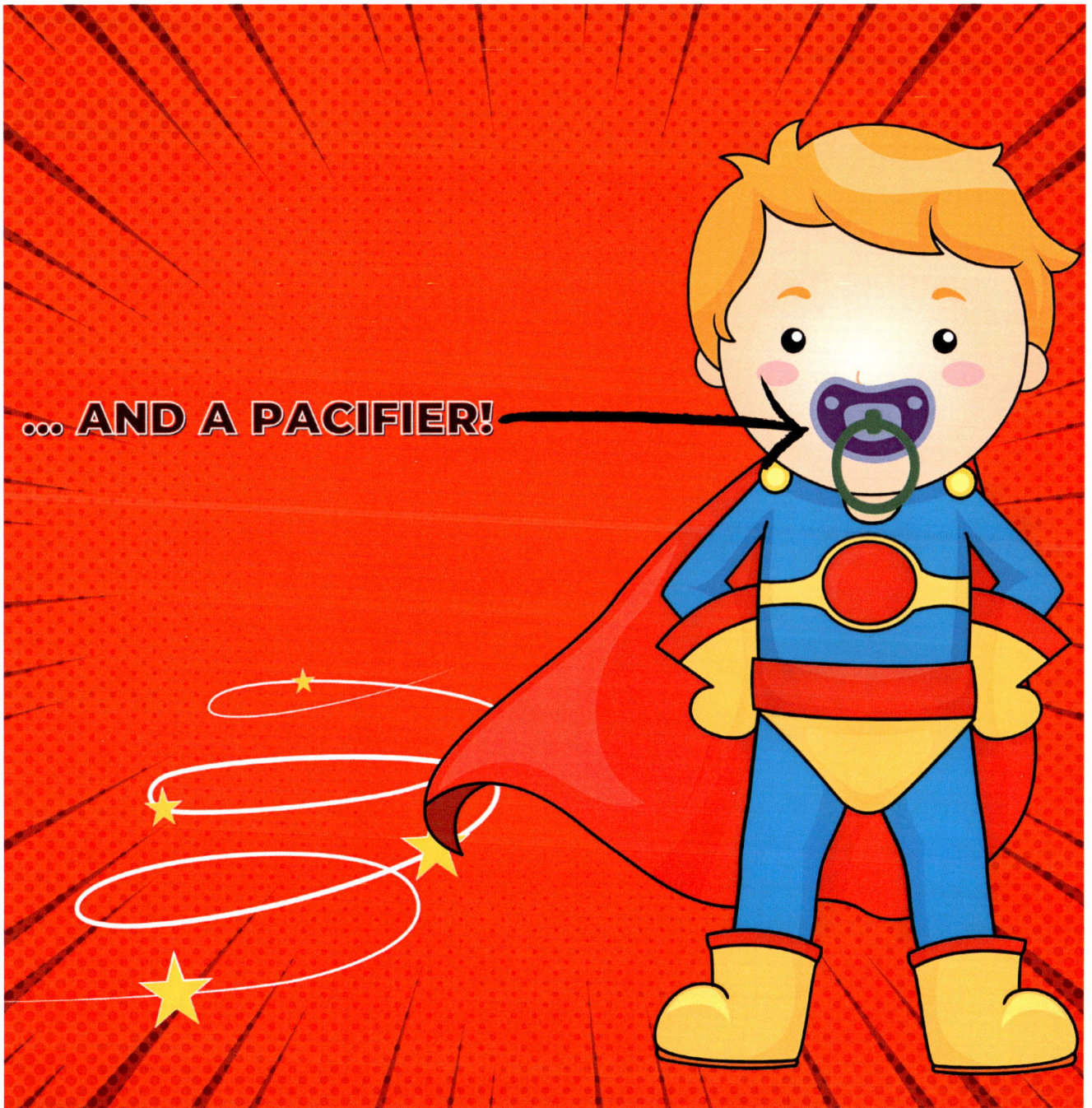

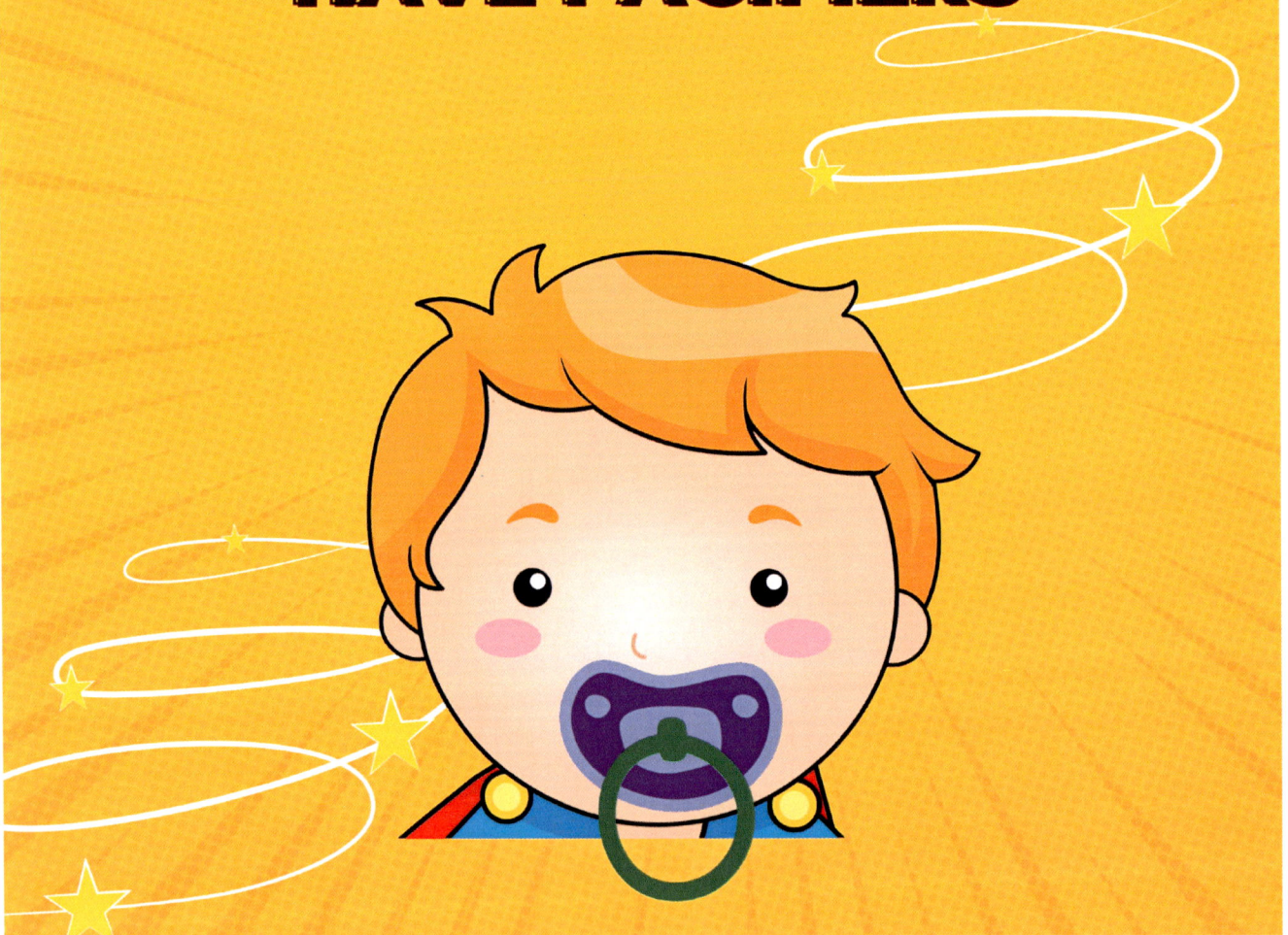

JAMES IS FAIRLY SURE SUPERHEROS DON'T HAVE PACIFIERS

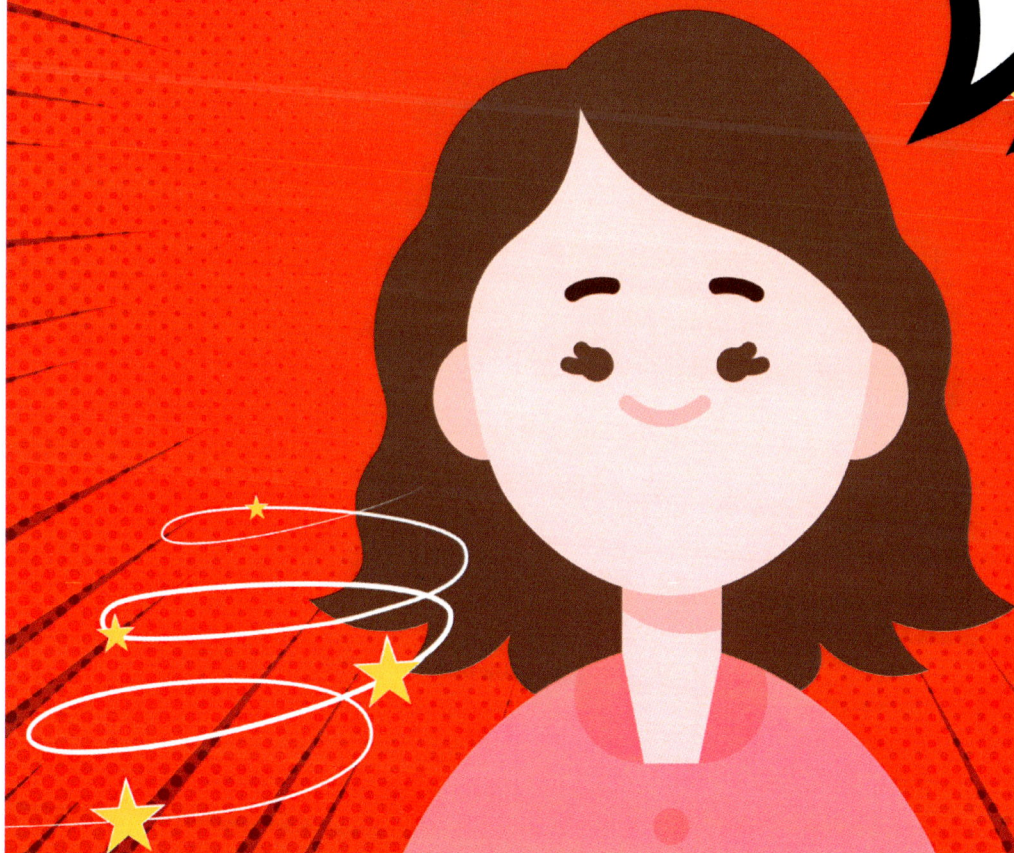

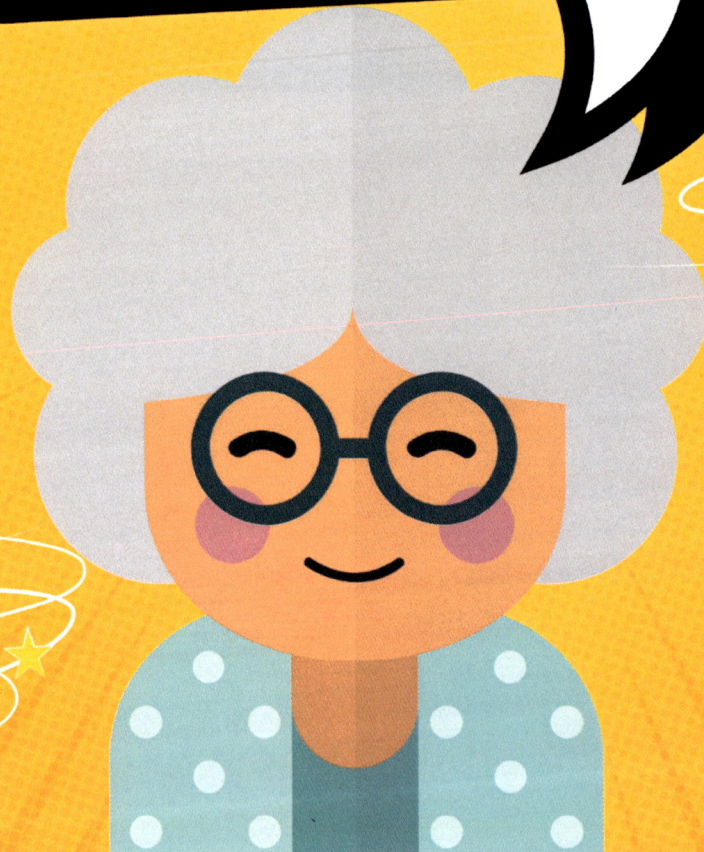

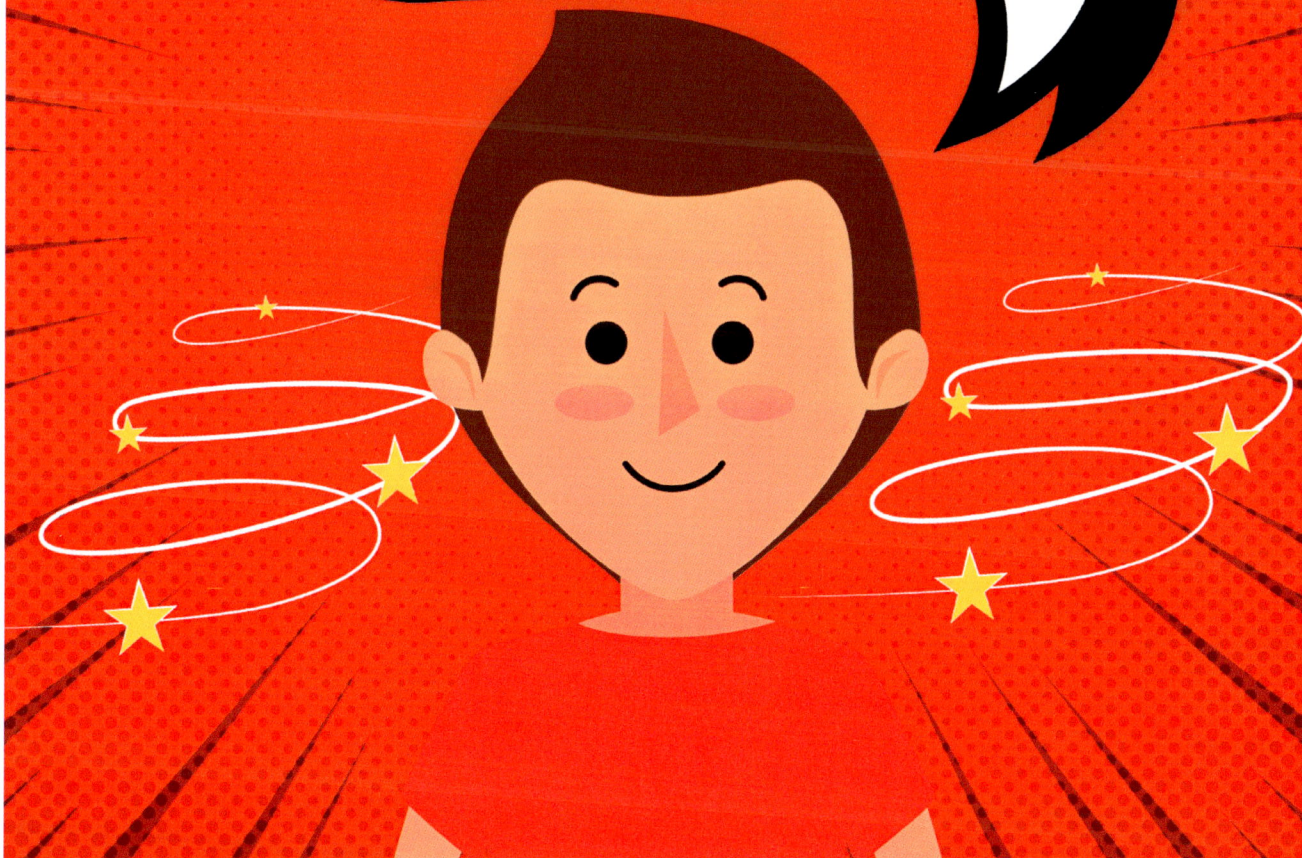

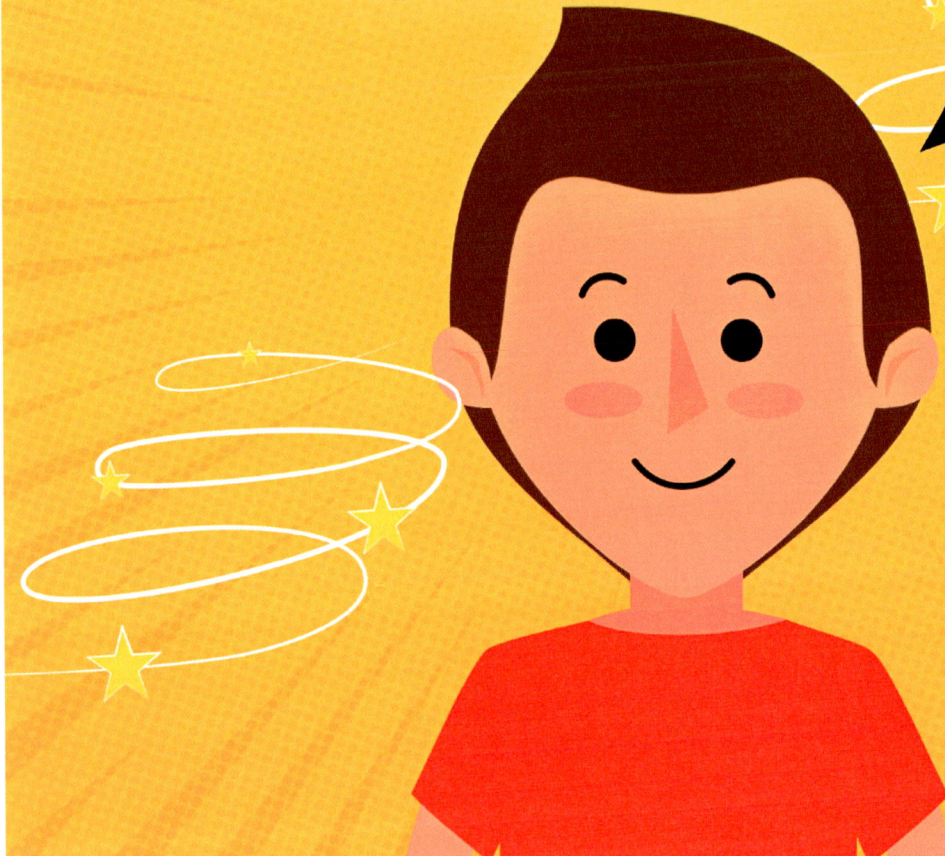

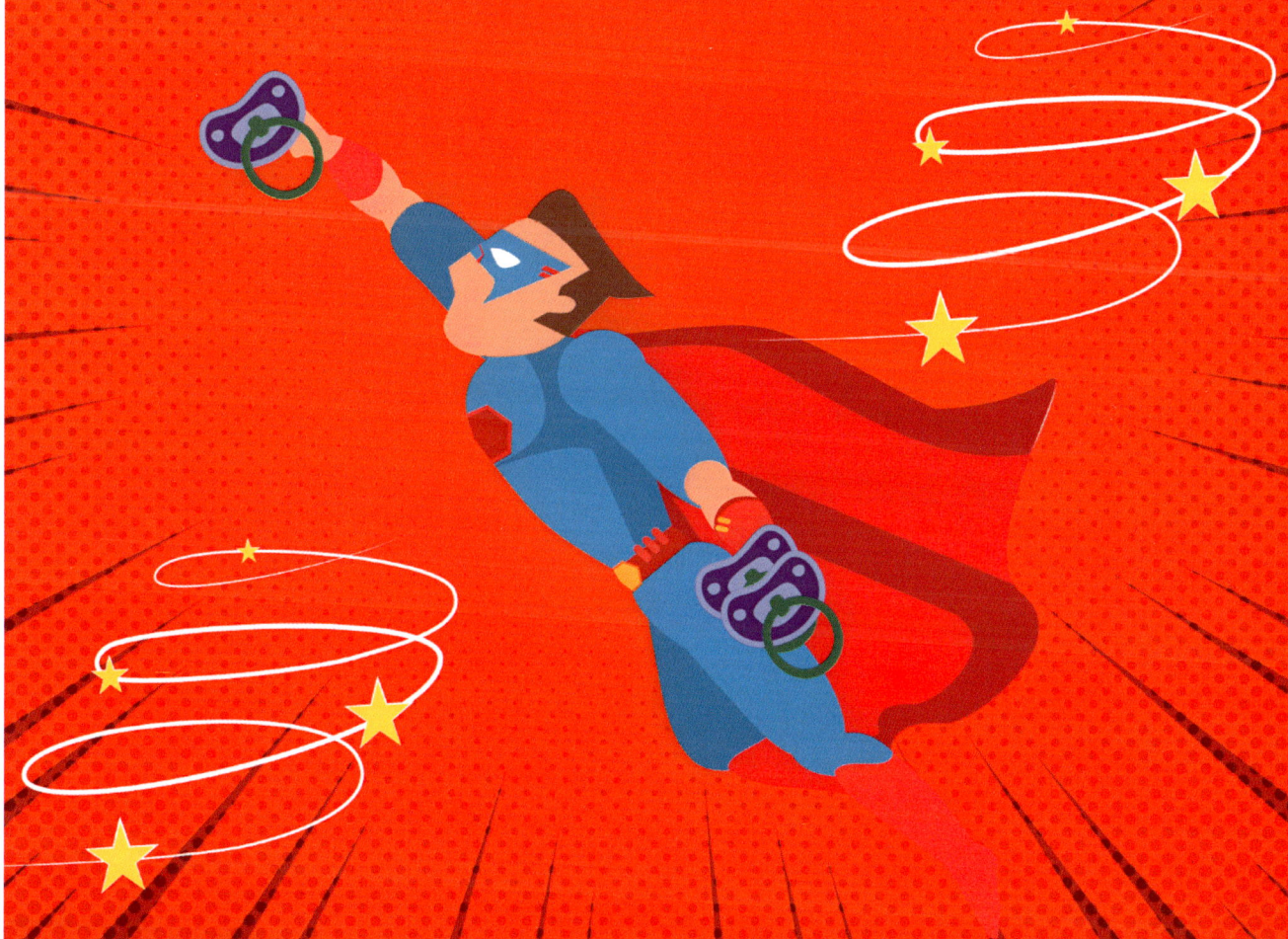

HE COLLECTS UP ALL THE PACIFIERS THE BIG KIDS DON'T NEED AND GIVES THEM TO THE BABIES TO STOP THEM CRYING

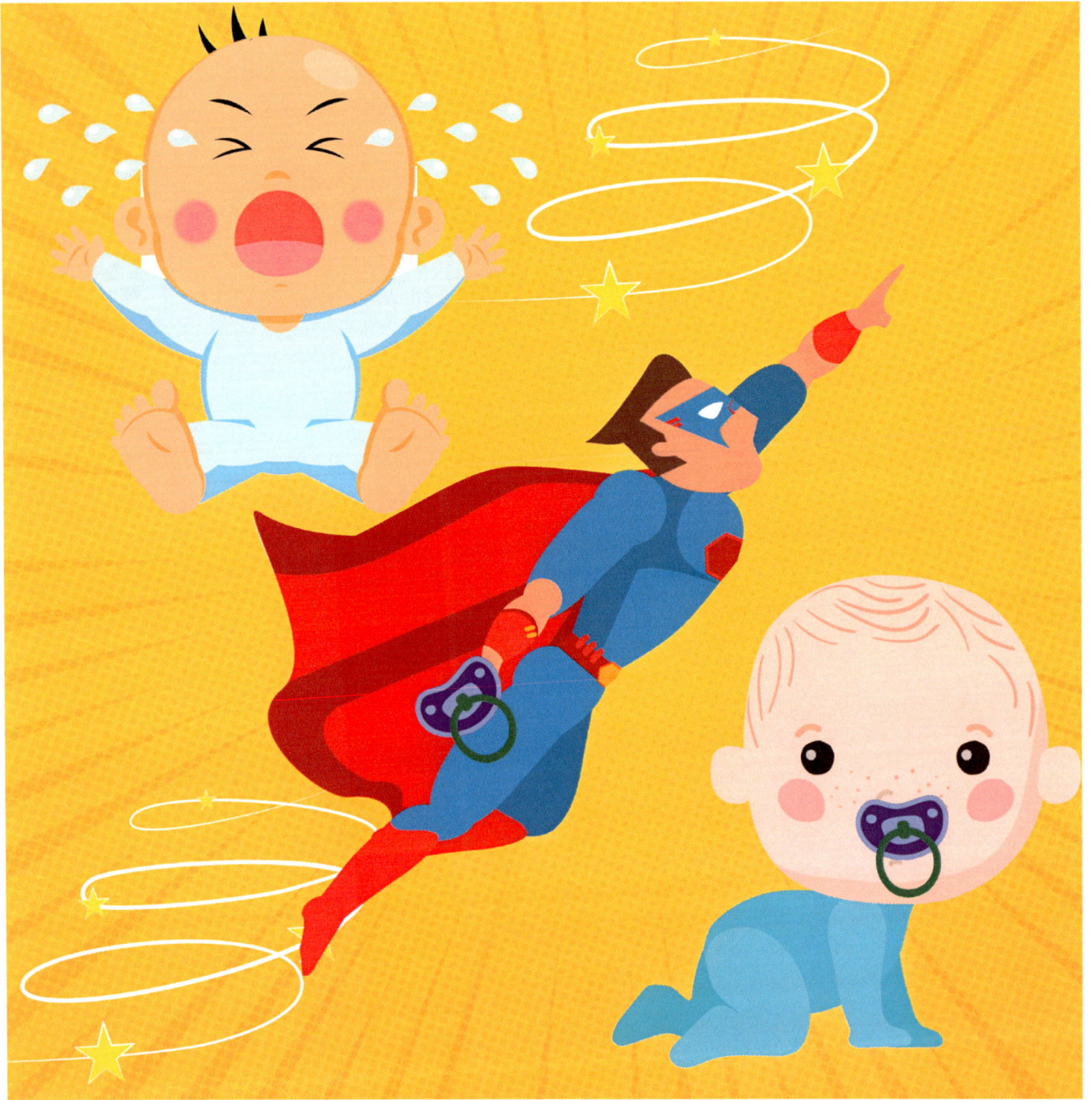

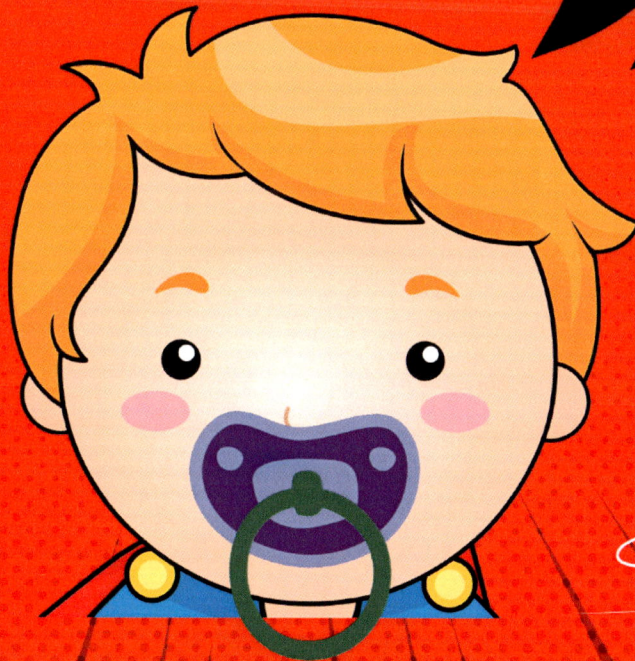

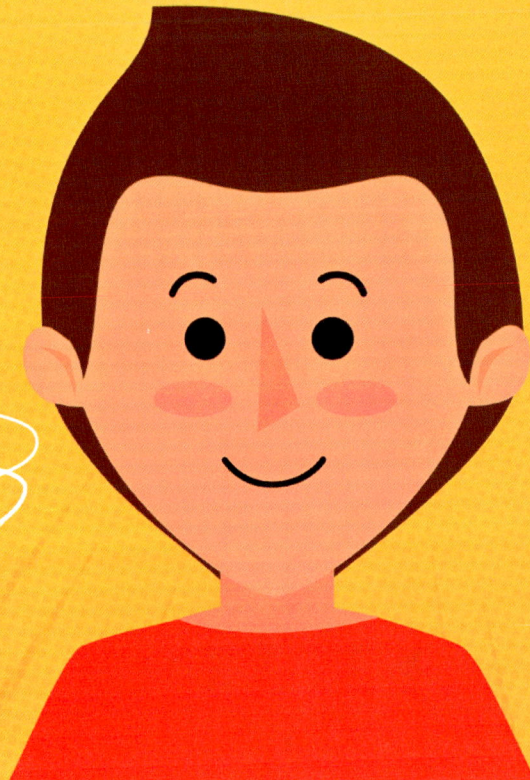

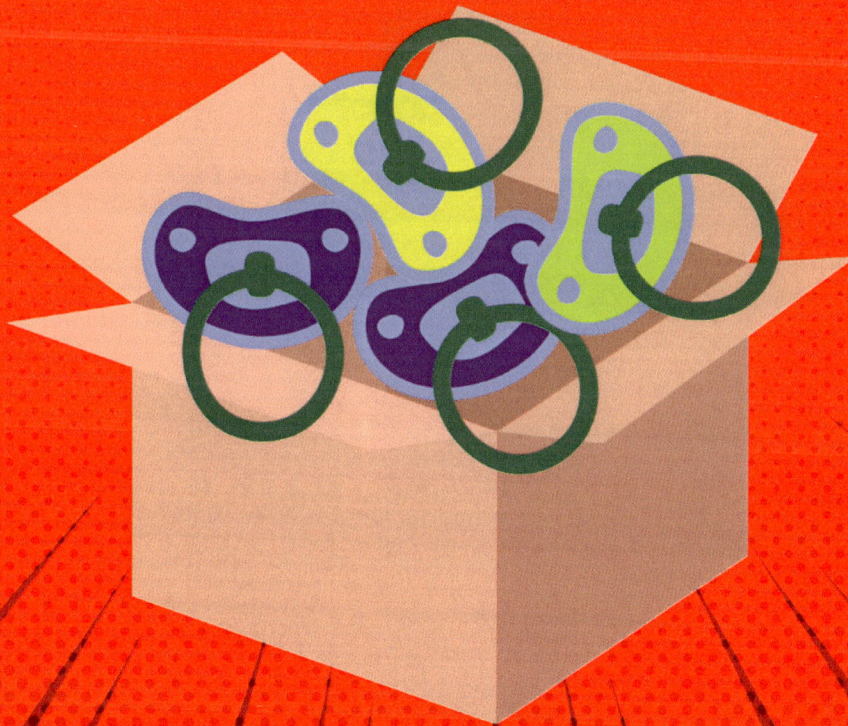

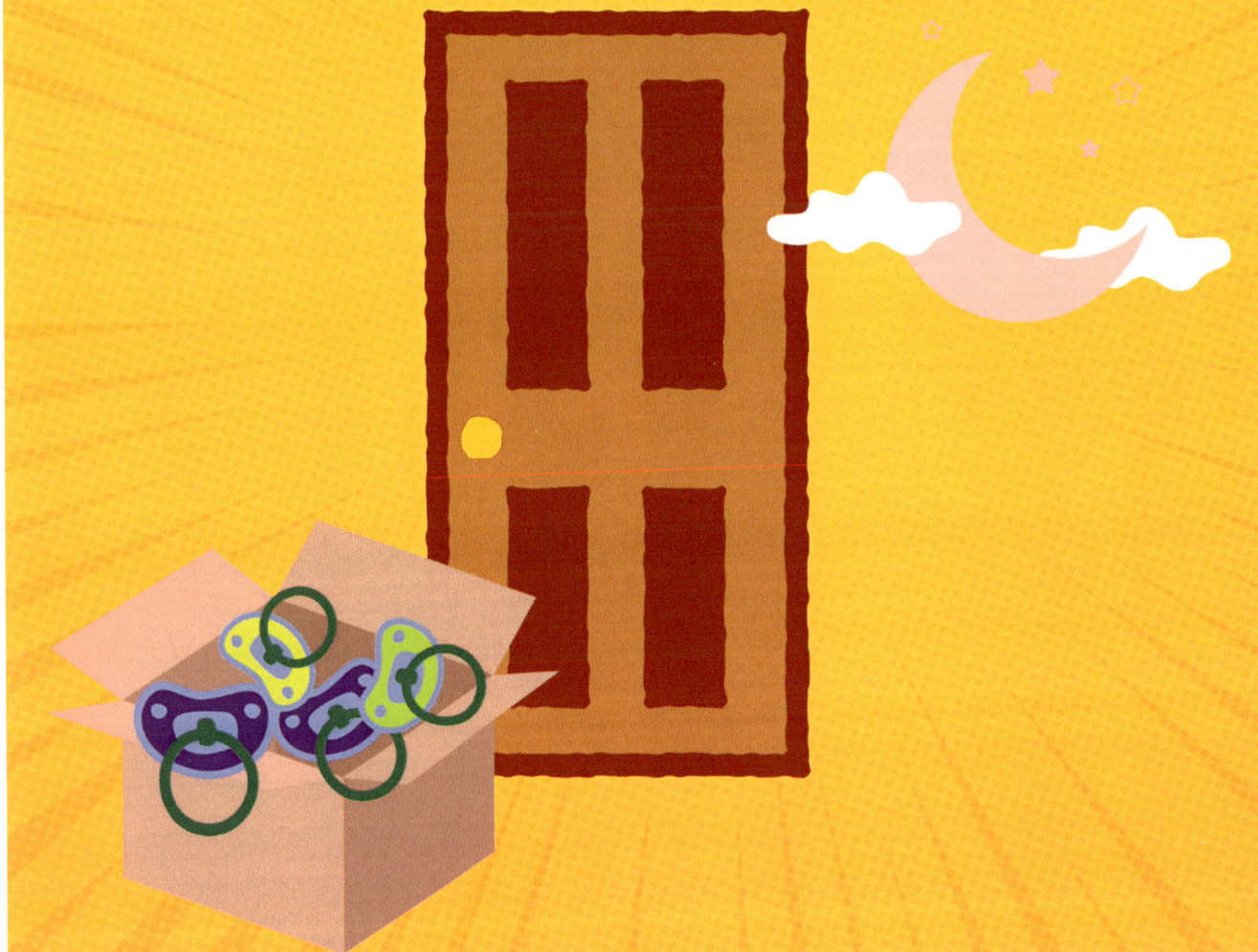

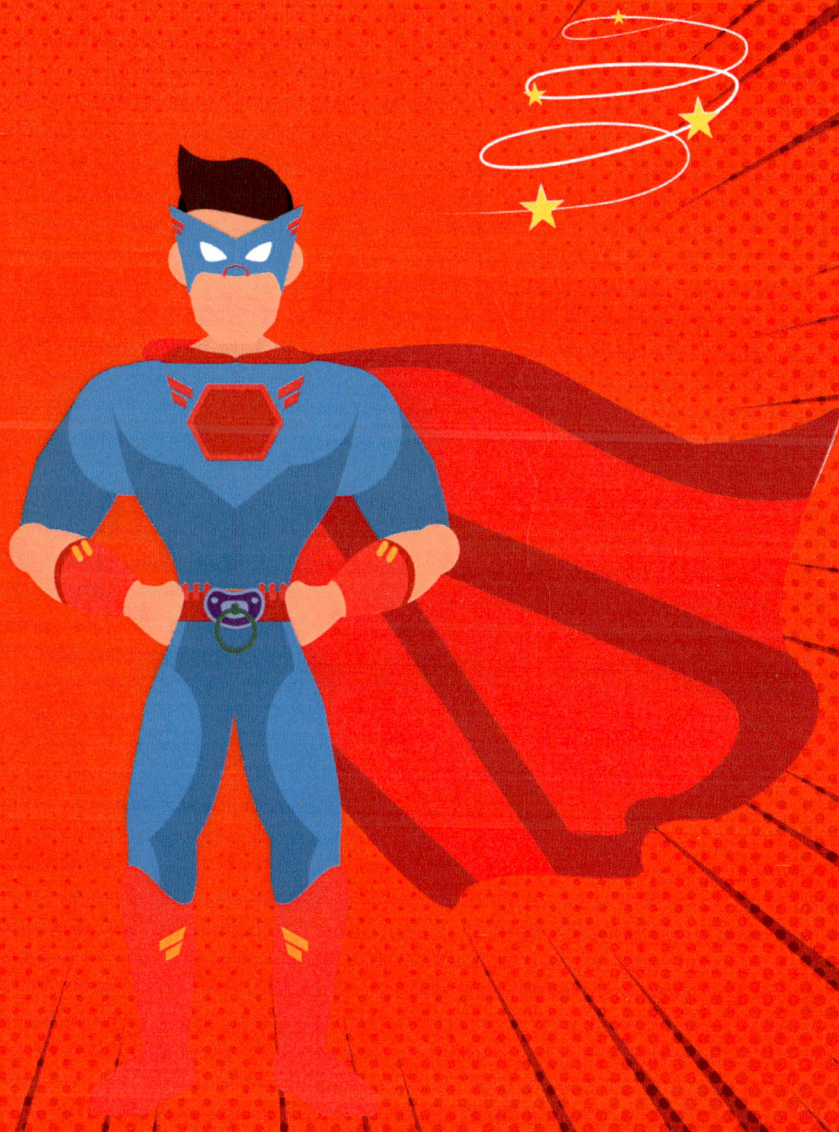
THE MAXIFIER ARRIVES IN THE MIDDLE OF THE NIGHT

THE MAXIFIER IS SO PLEASED WITH THE BOX OF PACIFIERS HE LEAVES AN EXTRA SPECIAL PRESENT FOR JAMES

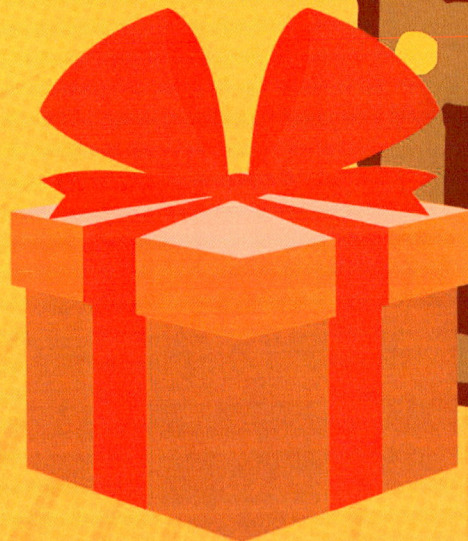

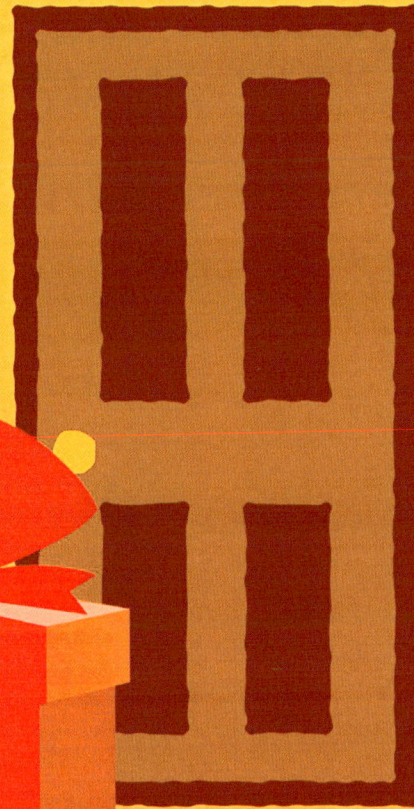

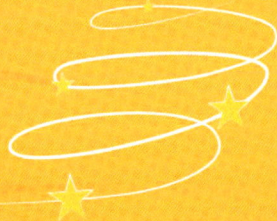

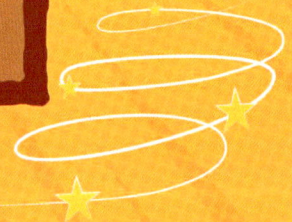

THE MAXIFIER HAS LEFT A NEW SUPERHERO CLOAK FOR JAMES

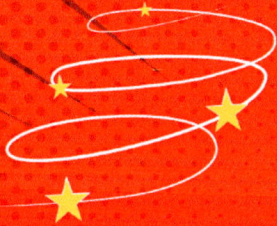

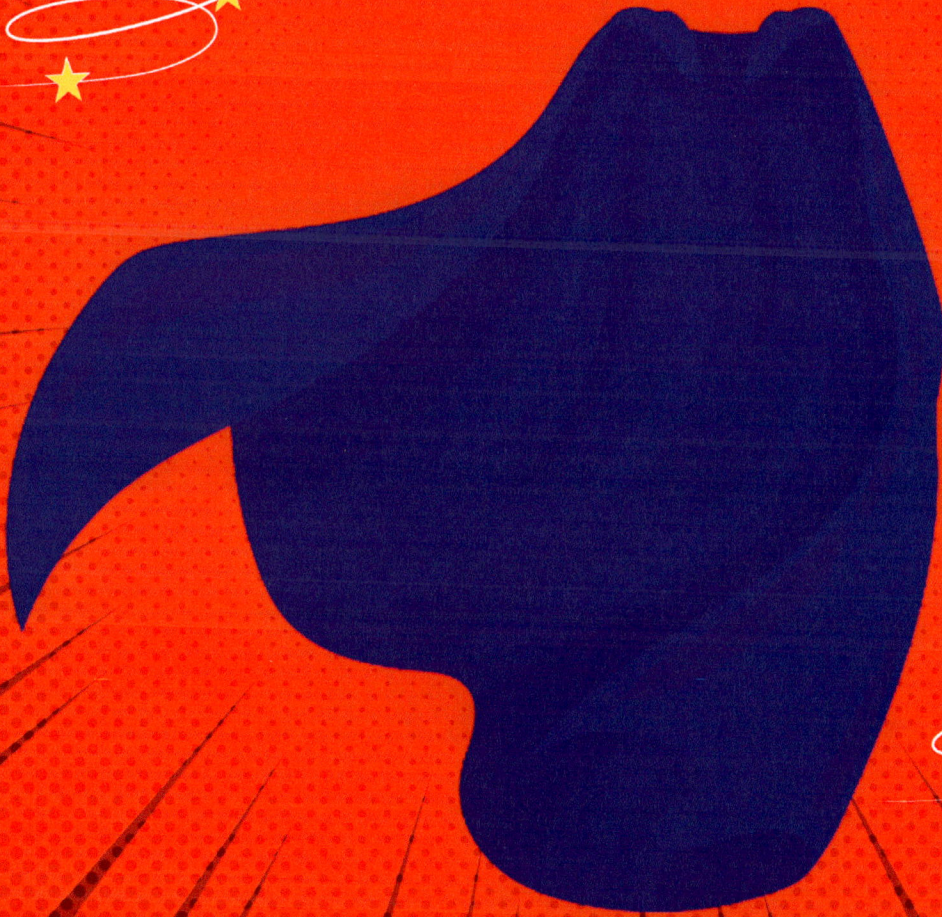

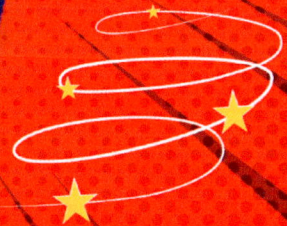

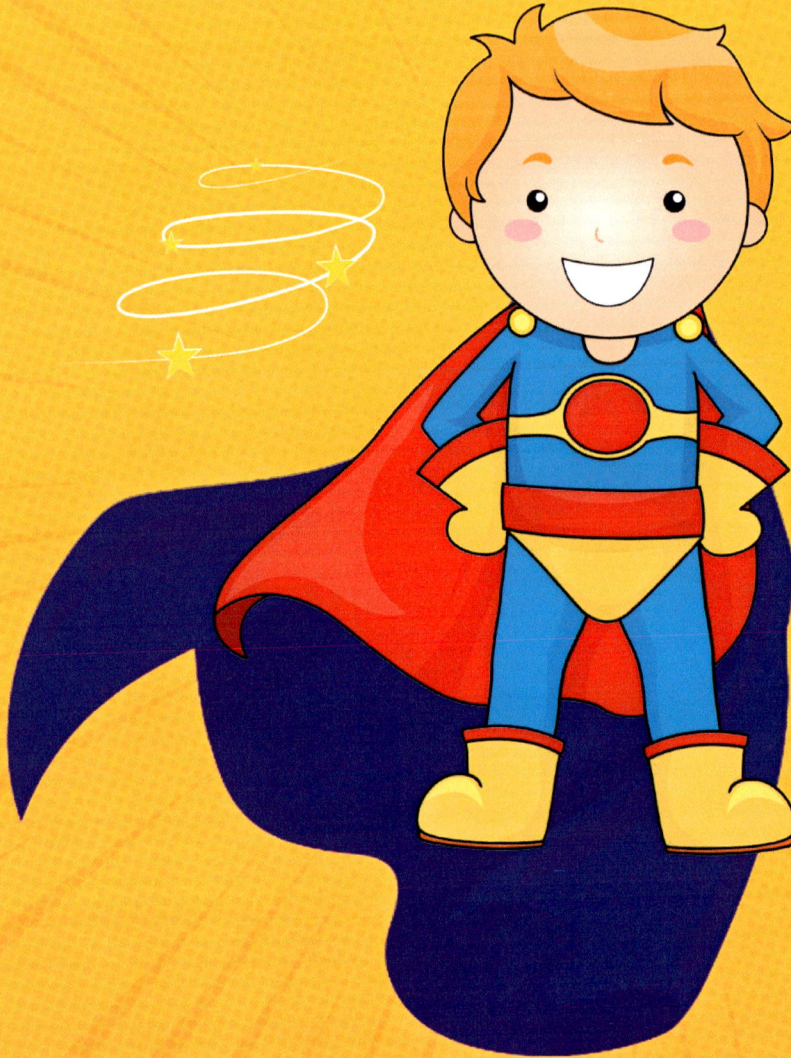
JAMES IS SO HAPPY HE WEARS BOTH CLOAKS

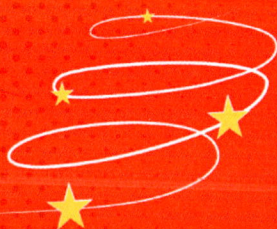

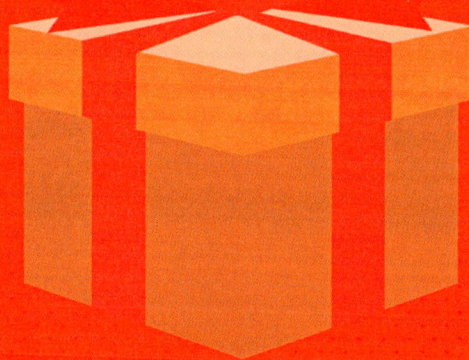

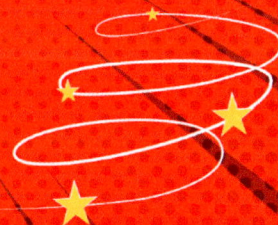

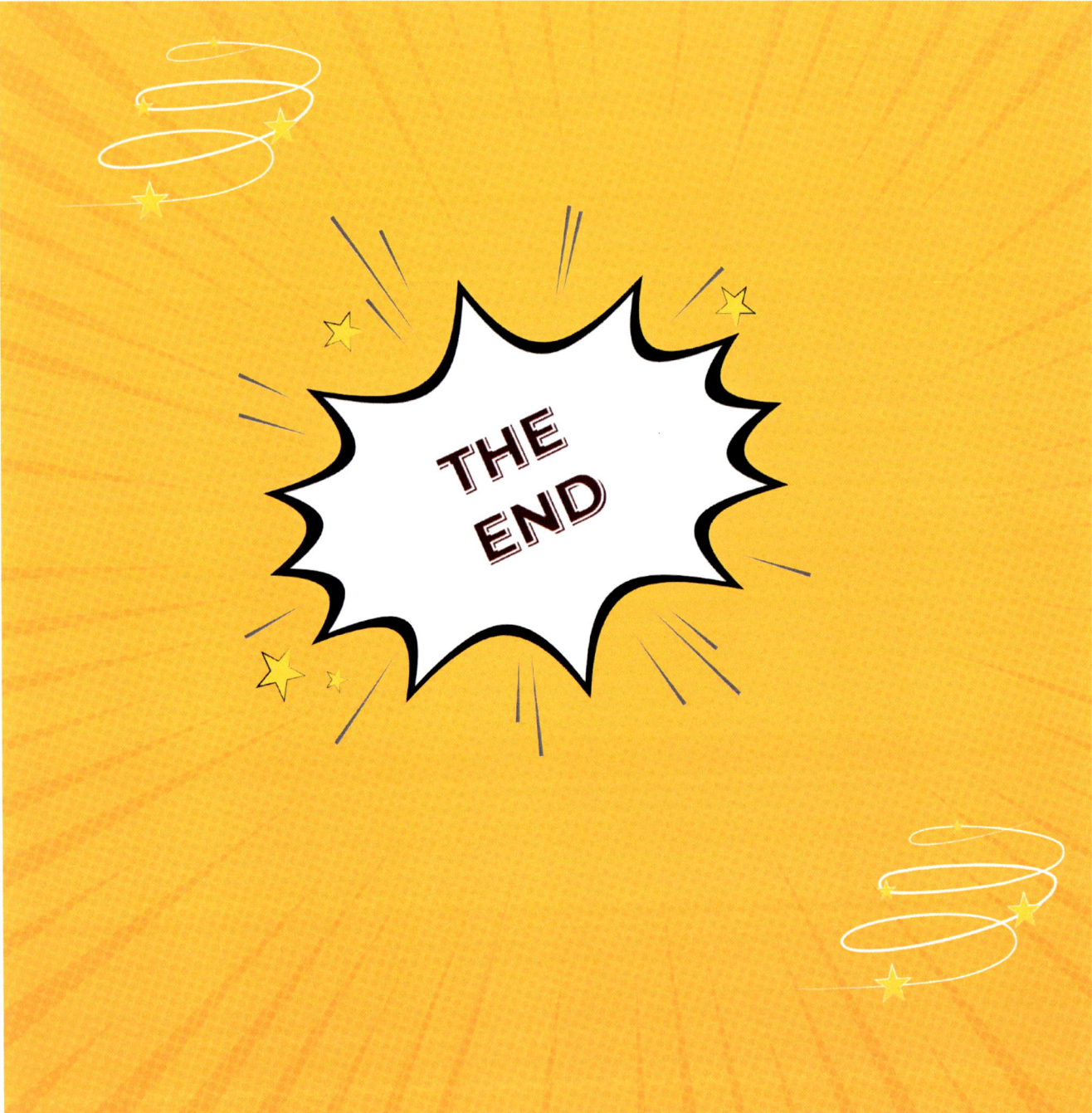

Made in United States
Orlando, FL
23 March 2025